GLUTEN FREE COOKBOOK

Let Food Be Thy Medicine

And

Medicine Thy Food

NICOLE TAMMY

Copyright © 2016   Nicole Tammy

All rights reserved. No part of this publication may be reproduced or distributed in any form or by any means, electronic or mechanical, or stored in a database or retrieval system, without prior written permission from the publisher.

Content

Introduction

1. Our Favorite Gluten-Free Pizza Dough; Page 1
2. Carrot Cake (Gluten & Dairy-Free); Page 5
3. Easy Gluten-Free Hushpuppies Recipe; Page 7
4. Gluten Free Waffles; Page 8
5. Gluten Free Flour Tortillas; Page 9
6. Gluten Free Crepes; Page 11
7. Gluten Free Sponge Cake; Page 12
8. German Pancake Gluten Free; Page 15
9. Gluten Free Cauliflower Cheddar Pancakes; Page 17
10. Gluten-Free Belgian Waffles with Buttermilk Syrup; Page 18
11. Lemon, Lavender & Honey Spa Party with Gluten-Free Lemon Cake Recipe; Page 19
12. Gluten-Free Chocolate Chip Cookies; Page 20
13. Gluten Free Stuffing; Page 21
14. Gluten Free Crepes; Page 23
15. Gluten Free Snickerdoodles Recipe; Page 24
16. Sandwich Bread (Gluten-Free Recipe); Page 26
17. Gluten-Free Peach Upside Down Cake; Page 28
18. Gluten Free Oatmeal Chocolate Chip Cookies; Page 30
19. Gluten-Free Banana Bread; Page 31
20. Gluten Free Blondies; Page 32
21. Egg Fast Recipe | Eggs Florentine; Page 34

22. Savory Vegetable Crumble (Vegan and Gluten Free); Page 36
23. Gluten Free Pumpkin Pie Hand Pies; Page 38
24. Gluten free super-fast sweet potato "steaks"; Page 40
25. Gluten-Free Apple-Spice Muffins; Page 41
26. Gluten Free Banana Pancakes; Page 42
27. Healthy Chocolate Crepes {Gluten and Grain Free}; Page 43
28. Gluten Free Lemon Chicken Chinese-Style; Page 45
29. Gluten Free Coconut Cream Cheesecake; Page 47
30. Gluten-free potato croquettes; Page 49

Introduction

My kitchen philosophy is simple, real, budget friendly, efficient, and family friendly. When it comes to the meals in this book, real food is at the heart of the recipes. I don't make a lot of fuss with most meals because I want to spend time with my family after school and on the weekends. I like to premake everything I can to help with efficiency. I premake sauce and stocks, and I even freeze meals along with the marinade so I can just thaw and cook! For this reason, I've included many make-ahead meals and tips on saving time.

My view of recipes is that they give me great ideas to play with. So please, use my recipes as a base ä joining off points" to create your own meals and your own flavor. Get creative! People have been gluten free for years. Take regular recipes and ask yourself what you can change to make them allergy-friendly. Yes, maybe you can't make the gluten filled crust, but the seasoning and sauce will definitely work effectively.

Get the taste & texture you remember from your pre-gluten free days with the added health benefits of whole grain flours, limited starches, lower sugar, and real, whole foods! The Gluten Free Cookbook helps bring your family back to the table, food allergies and all!

Our Favorite Gluten-Free Pizza Dough

In this recipe, we suggest you let your dough ferment for at least 24 hours before baking it. Honestly, the flavors deepen the longer you let it rest, so we generally make our dough on a Wednesday for Friday pizza night. When we make our pizza dough, we usually use 150 grams of our AP blend and 150 grams of our grain-free blend. Since we haven't told you the formula for that one yet, we made this pizza with 300 grams of our AP blend. It's still great. (But if you have any raw buckwheat flour on hand, try at least 100 grams of that in place of the AP.) Play with the flours you have on hand to make this yours.

- ¾ teaspoon active dry yeast
- 1 teaspoon sugar (or honey)
- 225 grams (about one cup) warm water (about 110°)
- 300 grams (about 2¼ cups) gluten-free girl all-purpose flour blend
- 6 grams (1½ teaspoons) psyllium husk
- 8 grams (1 teaspoon) sea salt
- 1 teaspoon olive oil

Instruction: Proof the yeast. Whisk together the yeast, sugar, and warm water, gently, in a small bowl. Let the yeasty water sit for at least 15 minutes. If the water is blooming with small bubbles and starting to smell yeasty, you have active yeast. Make the dough. Combine the two flours, the psyllium, and the salt in the bowl of a stand mixer with the paddle attachment. Whirl them up. With the mixer running on low, pour in the oil, then the yeasty water, very slowly. The dough will feel soft and pliable but softer and wetter than a typical gluten dough. (Try to mimic the texture of a creamy porridge.) Turn the mixer onto medium and let it run for a few more moments. Turn off the mixer and scrape down the sides of the bowl with a rubber spatula. Let the dough rise. Cover the bowl with plastic wrap and let it sit in a warm place for 1 hour. Then, put the dough in the refrigerator and let it sit overnight. Prepare to bake. The next day, pull the dough out of the refrigerator 1 hour before you intend to roll it. Divide the dough into 2 balls. Put one dough ball between 2 lightly greased pieces of parchment paper. Roll out the dough until it is about 12 inches across. Take the top piece of parchment paper off the dough. Curl up the edges of the dough, about 1/2 inch to 1 inch, all the way around the circle. Take a fork and gently crimp those edges onto the dough to seal them. Put the parchment paper back onto the dough. Put one hand under the bottom parchment paper, the other on top, and flip the dough. With slightly wet fingertips, make little indentations around the edges of the dough. Dock the pizza by making fork marks over the dough evenly. Transfer the dough to a baking sheet. Gently lift the edges of the dough to make sure no part of it is sticking to the parchment paper.

Repeat with the remaining dough ball.

Pre-bake the pizza dough. Heat the oven to 450°. Put the baking sheets in the oven—one on the lower rack and one in the middle. Bake until the tops of the doughs and the edges feel set, about 20 minutes. This will steam the water out of the doughs and give you a great dough for baking. Take the pizza doughs out of the oven.

Heat the oven higher. Bump up the temperature of the oven to as high as your oven will go. (Ours stops at 550°.) If you have a baking stone in the oven, that will generate even more heat in the oven.

Top the pizza. Top the pizza crusts with a drizzle of oil and any toppings you wish. This pizza was simply olive oil, tomato sauce, Parmesan cheese, sliced red peppers, and pepperoni.

Finish baking the pizza. Put the pizza in the oven when it's truly hot, then watch it. Wait until the cheese bubbles, then turn on the broiler at the end. Watch it closely. Don't let it burn. But get it to just before that point.

Voila! Pizza

Makes 2 (12-inch) pizza crusts

Feel like playing? Of course, you could use any flours you wish here, based on what works in your kitchen. Think of the psyllium husk here as just a touch more flour in the mix. It binds everything together beautifully without the gumminess (and for some, intestinal upset) of the gums. However, if you can't use psyllium, you could try finely ground flaxseed meal instead. But stick with this ratio. This ratio of flours to yeast to salt to psyllium to oil to water has worked for us every time. It's pizza dough.

Carrot Cake (Gluten & Dairy-Free)

Total Time: 60 minutes

Yield: two-layer 6" round cake, or 9x9" square cake

Ingredients

- 1 cup all-purpose gluten-free flour blend
- 1 tsp baking soda
- ½ tsp baking powder
- ½ tsp salt
- 1 tsp ground cinnamon
- ½ cup sugar (raw organic)
- ½ cup applesauce
- 1 egg
- 1 tsp vanilla extract
- ½ cup dairy free yogurt
- ¾ cup carrots, finely grated

Instructions

Preheat oven to 350 degrees F. Grease and flour a 9 x 9" pan or two round 6" cake pans.

Mix flour, baking soda, baking powder, salt and cinnamon in a small bowl, set aside.

Grate or process your carrots until fine. Measure and be sure you have ¾ cup carrots after processing. Set aside.

In a large bowl, whisk together the yogurt and egg.

Mix in sugar, applesauce and vanilla until smooth.

Add dry ingredients to wet mixture and mix until well combined.

Fold in carrots until evenly mixed.

Pour into your prepared cake pans and bake for 35-45 minutes until slightly golden brown and a toothpick inserted in the center comes out clean.

Let the cake sit in the pans for 5 minutes.

After 5 minutes remove and cool on a wire rack.

When cake is cooled, frost with your favorite dairy-free frosting (cream cheese is the best)!

Chill in the refrigerator until ready to serve!

Easy Gluten-Free Hushpuppies Recipe
Ingredients:

- 2 eggs
- ½ C sugar
- 1 onion, finely chopped
- ½ C Corn or rice flour
- ½ C gluten-free cornmeal
- Salt and pepper to taste

Instructions

Combine eggs, sugar, and onions in a large bowl.

Combine dry ingredients in a smaller bow, and add to egg mixture.

Heat deep fryer or a kettle of oil at least two inches deep over medium-high heat.

Once oil reaches 350-375°, drop hushpuppy dough in by heaping teaspoonful.

Turn once, if necessary (sometimes they roll themselves), once the bottom has become golden-brown.

Remove from oil onto paper towels to drain grease.

Serve with hushpuppy dipping sauce.

Gluten Free Waffles

Ingredients

- 3 cups Gluten Free Flour Blend
- ¾ cup ground flax
- 1 Tbsp. Cane sugar
- 1 tsp. sea salt
- 5 tsp. gluten-free baking powder
- 4 eggs, beaten
- ½ cup melted butter or coconut oil
- 1 tsp. gluten-free vanilla
- 2½ cups milk

Instruction:

In a large bowl mix dry ingredients together. Add all liquid ingredients and mix until smooth. It the batter sits for a while it will get thicker, add more milk if needed. Bake in a waffle iron. Serve immediately or cool on a rack and freeze.

Gluten Free Flour Tortillas
Ingredients:
- 1¾ cups (245 g) all-purpose gluten-free flour, plus more for sprinkling (I used Better Batter)
- 35 grams (about ¼ cup) Expandex modified tapioca starch* (or replace with an equal amount of tapioca starch/flour)
- 1½ teaspoons baking powder
- 1 teaspoon (6 g) kosher salt
- 4½ tablespoons (54 g) vegetable shortening
- ¾ cup (6 ounces) warm water (about 85°F)

In a large bowl, place the all-purpose flour, Expandex, baking powder, and salt, and whisk to combine. Add the vegetable shortening and toss it in the dry ingredients. With the tines of a large fork, break up the shortening into small pieces about the size of small peas. Create a well in the center of the mixture, and add most of the water. Mix to combine. The dough will come together and be thick. If there are any crumbly bits, add the remaining water by the teaspoonful. Knead the dough together and press it into a ball, cover with a moist tea towel, and allow to sit for about 20 minutes. The dough will stiffen a bit as it absorbs more of the water.

Heat a 10- or 12-inch cast-iron skillet over medium-high heat. Divide the dough into five pieces. Begin with one piece of dough, and cover the rest with a moist tea towel to prevent them from drying out. On a lightly floured surface, with a rolling pin, roll out the first piece of dough until it is 1/8 inch thick. Cut out as many rounds as you can (should be three or four) with a 6- or 8-inch metal cake cutter. Stack the raw tortillas on top of one another, dusting lightly with flour between them, if necessary, to prevent them from sticking. Gather the scraps and set them aside. Repeat with the remaining pieces of dough, including gathering and rerolling all of the scraps together.

Once all the tortillas have been rolled out and cut, place them one at a time in the center of the hot skillet and cook on one side until bubbles begin to appear on the top surface and the tortilla darkens in color a bit on the underside (about 45 seconds). Flip the tortilla over with a wide spatula, and cook on the other side until more bubbles form and the tortilla darkens on the underside (about another 45 seconds). Remove the tortilla from the pan, place on a moist tea towel, and cover gently. Repeat with the remaining tortillas.

If you don't plan to use the tortillas right away, place them, still wrapped in the towel, in a plastic bag to seal in the moisture. Use within a few hours.

Gluten Free Crepes

Ingredients:
- 1½ cups Gluten Free Flour Blend
- 3 eggs
- 2 Tbsp. melted butter
- 1¼ cup milk

Instruction:
Blend all ingredients together until smooth. Preheat a heavy frypan and lightly grease with butter. Pour 2 - 3 tablespoons (depending on the size of your pan) onto pan and tip and swirl to coat with a thin layer. As the batter sets gently lift edge with a spatula, when crepe is lightly brown turn to brown the other side. (I usually turn with my fingers). I have found the key to having them not stick is having the pan hot enough. Stack crepes on a plate. Fill as desired.

Gluten Free Sponge Cake

Ingredients:

- 4 eggs (200g, out of shell), separated
- ¾ cup (150g) granulated sugar
- 1/2 teaspoon cream of tartar (or 1 tablespoon freshly squeezed lemon juice)
- 10 tablespoons (88g) Basic Gum Free Gluten Free Flour Blend (58g superfine white rice flour + 19g potato starch + 11 g tapioca starch/flour)
- 2 tablespoons (18g) cornstarch (or try arrowroot)
- ¼ teaspoon kosher salt
- 1 teaspoon pure vanilla extract

Directions:

Preheat your oven to 350°F. Grease a 9-inch round cake pan* well and set it aside.

*Alternatively, multiply all of the ingredients in this recipe by 150% or 1.5. Follow the recipe instructions as written, but divide the batter between two 8-inch cake pans. Bake them for about 25 minutes or until the cakes have begun to pull away from the sides of the pan and a toothpick comes out mostly clean, or with a few moist crumbs attached.

In the bowl of your stand mixer fitted with the paddle attachment (or a large bowl with a hand mixer), place the egg yolks and 1/2 cup (100 g) sugar, and beat on medium-high speed until pale yellow. Sift the flour blend, cornstarch and salt into the egg yolk mixture, and beat until well-combined. Transfer the egg yolk mixture to a small bowl and set aside.

Clean out the mixer bowl very well, and place the egg whites and cream of tartar or lemon juice in the bowl, fitted with the whisk attachment. Beat the egg whites on medium-high speed until soft peaks form. Add the remaining 1/4 cup (50 g) sugar, and beat until glossy, stiff (but not dry) peaks form. With the mixer on medium speed, slowly pour the egg yolk mixture and the vanilla into the egg white mixture, and beat until just combined. The mixture should be smooth and glossy.

Pour the batter into the prepared pan, and spread into an even layer. Place in the center of the preheated oven and bake until the cake has begun to pull away from the sides of the pan and a toothpick comes out mostly clean, or with a few moist crumbs attached (about 35 minutes). Allow the cake to cool in the pan for about 10 minutes before transferring to a wire rack to cool completely.

Serving Suggestion:

Cool the cake completely, then wrap it tightly and freeze for 30 minutes. Unwrap and slice the cake in half horizontally, fill with fresh whipped cream or 7-minute frosting and a layer of sliced strawberries. Top with the other half of the cake, more whipped cream or frosting and another layer of sliced strawberries. Chill for about 2 hours before serving.

German Pancake Gluten Free

Prep time 10 mins
Cook time 20 mins
Total time 30 mins

Ingredients

- 3 Large Eggs
- ½ Cup of Whole Milk
- ½ Cup Gluten-Free All Purpose Flour
- ⅛ Tsp. Salt
- 2 Tbsp. Unsalted Butter
- Fresh Lemon
- Powdered Sugar

Instructions:

Place the butter in the center of a 10-inch cast iron skillet and place it in the oven. Now preheat oven to 375 degrees Fahrenheit.

In a large bowl, whisk together the eggs and milk. Next, whisk in the flour and salt until combined.

Once the oven is pre-heated, open the oven and carefully pull out the rack with the hot skillet. Slowly pour the batter in the middle of the melted butter. Gently push the rack back in and close the oven door. Bake the pancake for 25 minutes or until golden brown around the edges. If your oven cooks unevenly rotate the pan half way through baking.

Cut the pancake into wedges and serve immediately. Butter the pancake and top with powdered sugar and lemon juice.

Gluten Free Cauliflower Cheddar Pancakes

Ingredients

- 1 bag riced cauliflower, or a head of cauliflower riced
- ¾ cup Vermont cheddar cheese, shredded
- 1 large leek, sliced
- 3 tablespoons grated parmesan cheese
- ½ teaspoon salt
- 3 tablespoons olive oil
- ¼ cup gluten free flour blend
- ½ cup almond milk, (or regular milk if you have it.)
- ¼ teaspoon cayenne pepper (optional)
- Garnish with sour cream and scallion

Instructions

Start heating oil in a pan on medium high heat.

Add riced cauliflower, cheese, salt, flour, leek and milk to a bowl and mix well.

Test oil temperature by dropping a drip of water into the pan. If it sizzles, it is ready.

Form patties.

Drop patties into the hot oil.

Cook until golden on each side, about 3-4 minutes per side.

Remove from heat and put each patty onto a plate covered in paper towels (to absorb extra oil)

Serve with sour cream and scallions

Gluten-Free Belgian Waffles with Buttermilk Syrup

Ingredients:

- 4 large eggs, separated
- 3 C gluten-free all-purpose flour plus 1/4 tsp. xanthan gum OR Pamela's Products Baking & Pancake Mix
- 1 ½ C milk
- 4 T coconut oil
- ½ C butter
- ¾ C sugar
- ½ C buttermilk
- 1 tablespoon gluten-free vanilla
- 1 tablespoon aluminum-free baking soda

Instructions:

In a bowl, whip egg whites until stiff. In another bowl, mix gluten-free flour mix, egg yolks, milk and coconut oil together until there are no lumps. Fold in stiff egg whites and cook in preheated, greased Belgian waffle iron. For the buttermilk syrup, bring first butter, sugar and buttermilk to a boil. Remove from heat and add vanilla and baking soda. While you can use gluten-free all-purpose flour and xanthan gum, I highly recommend using the Pamela's Products Baking and Pancake Mix we did. The flavor is so delicious and definitely a step above the gluten-free all-purpose flours I've used. Whatever you choose to use, I hope you all love this recipe as much as my family and I do…

Lemon, Lavender & Honey Spa Party with Gluten-Free Lemon Cake Recipe

Ingredients:

- 2¼ C gluten-free all-purpose flour
- 1 tablespoon Real Salt
- 1 tablespoon baking powder
- 2/3 C coconut oil
- 1 1/3 C sugar
- 2½ T real lemon juice
- ½ C whole milk
- 3 large eggs

Instructions:

Preheat oven to 325°. Cream together wet ingredients. Slowly add in dry ingredients. Mix 1-2 minutes then pour into greased 9x13 pan. Bake 60 minutes or until a toothpick inserted in the center comes out clean.

Gluten-Free Chocolate Chip Cookies

- 2.5 cups of powdered sugar
- 1/2 Cup cocoa
- ½ tsp cinnamon
- ¼ tsp salt
- 3 egg whites
- 1 tsp vanilla extract
- 2 cups chocolatey.

Instruction:

1. Preheat the oven to 175 C. g Mix icing sugar, cocoa, cinnamon and salt. Stir in the whites, with a mixer, but do not beat! Just mix up the connections.
2. Stir in vanilla and chocolate. The dough will be liquid, spread it with a spoon on a baking sheet, leaving a 3 cm distance.
3. Bake 15 minutes, let cool on baking sheets for 10 minutes, then you can shift.

Gluten Free Stuffing

Prep time 10 mins
Cook time 50 mins
Total time 1 hour

Ingredients:
- 1 Loaf Gluten Free Bread
- ½ of an Onion
- 4 Cloves of Garlic
- 1 Celery Stock
- ¾ Cup Turkey or Chicken Stock
- 1 Teaspoon Basil
- ½ Teaspoon Salt (If using store bought stock you may not need to add any salt)
- ½ Teaspoon Pepper

Instructions:
Cut up the loaf of bread into ½ inch pieces, then place into a large mixing bowl.

Mince the onion, garlic and celery, then add to the bowl. Add the stock along with the basil and salt and pepper.

Mix until well combined.

Use the gluten free stuffing to stuff your turkey or chicken or Place the stuffing into a large lightly greased or parchment paper lined baking dish or onto a cookie sheet. Bake in the oven @ 350 F for 45-50 minutes, stirring a few times throughout.

Gluten Free Crepes

Serves 8

This is the perfect breakfast or brunch for a special morning, celebration, or just because. Light, fluffy, and wonderful!

Ingredients:

- 2 eggs
- 2 Teaspoon coconut oil, melted & cooled
- 1 Teaspoon honey or pure maple syrup
- 1 c. gluten free oat flour
- 1½ c. almond milk

Instructions:

Combine all ingredients in a blender. Blend on low speed until well combined, and smooth. Crepe batter will be a very thin consistency and easily pourable. Heat a skillet over medium high heat. Grease lightly with butter or cooking spray. Pour about 1/4 c. of crepe batter into the pan; twirl in a circular motion to coat evenly with batter. Let cook about thirty to sixty seconds, or until the edges of the batter bubble slightly, and it's easy to slide a spatula under the edge of the crepe. Flip crepe and cook another fifteen to thirty seconds. Remove from pan and stack on a plate.

Gluten Free Snickerdoodles Recipe

Ingredients:

- 1½ cups granulated cane sugar
- 1 cup shortening, butter or other non-dairy alternative (e.g. Earth Balance® Buttery Sticks/Shortening Sticks)
- 2 large eggs or egg substitute
- 2¾ cups Gluten Free All Purpose Flour
- 1 Teaspoon baking soda
- 2 Teaspoon cream of tartar
- ¼ Teaspoon salt
- 2 Teaspoon granulated cane sugar (optional)
- 2 Teaspoon cinnamon (optional)

Method:

Cream shortening and sugar until fluffy. Add eggs and beat until combined.

In a separate bowl, whisk dry ingredients together: All Purpose Flour; baking soda, cream of tartar and salt. Add to wet ingredient bowl and mix until thoroughly incorporated.

Cover tightly and refrigerate until cold, at least 2 hours.

Preheat oven to 400 F (static) or 375 F (convection).

Shape dough into 1-inch balls by rolling in the palms of your hands. Roll each ball in the sugar and cinnamon mixture. Place on a parchment-lined baking sheet and bake for 8-9 minutes, or until lightly browning and puffed.

Remove to cool on a wire rack; the cookies will sink slightly in the middle when cooled – this is completely normal.

Yield: approximately 3 dozen cookies.

Sandwich Bread (Gluten-Free Recipe)

Ingredients:

- 1 cup warm milk, (about 110°F)
- 1/4 cup sugar
- 2¼ teaspoons active dry yeast
- 2½ cups Gluten-Free Flour Blend
- 1 teaspoon salt
- ¼ cup Land O Lakes Butter, melted, cooled
- 2 Land O Lakes Eggs

Directions:

Combine milk, sugar and yeast in bowl; set aside 10 minutes.

Combine flour blend and salt in large stand mixer bowl; beat with stand mixer on low speed, gradually adding yeast mixture until well combined. Add butter and eggs; beat, scraping bowl occasionally, until well mixed. Increase speed to high; beat about 3 minutes or until batter is very smooth.

Cover, let rise in warm place 1 hour.

Grease 8x4-inch loaf pan. Stir dough; pour into pan, leveling top. Loosely cover with greased plastic food wrap; let rise 20-30 minutes or until just above top edge of pan.

Heat oven to 350°F.

Bake 42-50 minutes or until top is golden brown. Remove bread from pan; cool completely on cooling rack.

Recipe Tips

Gluten-Free Flour Blend: Combine 2 cups rice flour, 2/3 cup potato starch (do not use potato flour), 1/3 cup tapioca flour and 1 teaspoon xanthan gum. Use appropriate amount for recipe; store remainder in container with tight-fitting lid. Stir before using.

This recipe was developed using alternative flours and products labeled as "gluten-free." The best source for additional information is the ingredient listing on product packaging. Learn about gluten-free baking.

For easy storage and to increase shelf life - slice bread and package individually. Store in freezer and take out a slice at a time for fresh bread.

It is important to use potato starch not potato flour in the Gluten-Free Flour Blend.

Gluten-Free Peach Upside Down Cake

Recipe type: Dessert

Prep time: 10 mins

Cook time: 35 mins

Total time: 45 mins

A good Upside Down Cake is a thing of beauty. Beautiful, juicy peaches make this one both gorgeous and delicious.

Ingredients:

- About 2 teaspoons unsalted butter (or non-dairy butter equivalent)
- 2 peaches, peeled and sliced
- ⅓ cup dark brown sugar
- 1½ cups gluten-free all-purpose flour mix (Steve recommends a lighter gluten-free flour mix like he used; see notes. I'd use my Two-Ingredient Gluten-Free Flour Mix.)
- ½ teaspoon xanthan gum
- ¾ cup granulated sugar
- 1½ tsp baking powder
- 1 teaspoon cinnamon
- ½ teaspoon baking soda
- ½ teaspoon salt
- ¾ cup buttermilk (see notes for substitutions, including dairy-free option)

- 2 large eggs, at room temperature, slightly beaten
- ⅓ cup canola oil (or oil of choice)
- 1 teaspoon vanilla extract

Instructions:

Using butter, grease an 8 x 8 pan thoroughly (bottom and sides).

Sprinkle brown sugar on the bottom of the pan and top with the peach slices.

In a large bowl, combine gluten-free flour mix, xanthan gum, granulated sugar, baking powder, cinnamon, baking soda and salt.

Add the buttermilk, eggs, oil, and vanilla extract to your dry mixture. Whisk until combined.

Pour the cake batter over the peaches and brown sugar base.

Bake at 350 for about 35 minutes until a toothpick inserted into the center comes out clean.

Cool in the pan for 5 minutes. To loosen the cake, run a knife along the edges of the pan. Turn cake onto a wire rack to cool completely.

Gluten Free Oatmeal Chocolate Chip Cookies

- 1 cup butter at room temperature
- ½ cup cane sugar (or ½ cup white sugar + ½ cup brown sugar)
- 2 large eggs
- 4 tsp. Vanilla
- 2 cups Gluten Free Flour Blend
- 1 tsp. Baking soda
- ½ tsp. sea salt
- ¼ tsp xanthan gum
- 1 cup GF oatmeal
- 1½ cups milk chocolate chips

Cream together butter and sugar. Add eggs and vanilla and beat until light. Stir together flour, soda, salt and xanthan gum, add to batter and mix until well combined. Stir in oatmeal and chocolate chips. Refrigerate for one hour then shape dough into one inch balls and flatten with the palm of your hand on a cookie sheet. Bake at 350 degrees for 10 -12 minutes or until lightly browned. Cool on the pan for 5 minutes, transfer to a wire rack to cool completely. Yield: 2 1/2 doz.

Gluten-Free Banana Bread

Serves: 2 loaves

Ingredients:
- ½ cup butter
- 1½ cups sugar
- 2 cups gluten-free flour
- ½ tablespoon salt
- 1 cup sour cream
- 2 eggs, beaten
- 3 mashed bananas
- 1 tablespoon baking soda
- 1 tablespoon vanilla

Instructions:
Preheat oven to 300 degrees.

Grease and flour 2 bread pans.

Cream butter and sugar together.

Add eggs and bananas. Mix well.

Sift flour, salt, and baking soda together and add to the mixture.

Mix until well combined and then add vanilla.

Fold in the sour cream.

Bake at 300 degrees for 1 hour, or until a toothpick comes out clean.

Gluten Free Blondies

Prep time 10 mins

Cook time 30 mins

Total time 40 mins

serves: 9 blondies

Ingredients:

- 1 cup Gluten Free Flour (I used King Arthur Gluten-Free Flour)
- 1 cup light brown sugar, packed
- ½ cup butter, softened
- 1 large egg, room temperature
- 1 teaspoon vanilla extract
- ½ teaspoon baking soda
- ½ teaspoon salt
- 1 cup dark chocolate baking disks/chocolate chips

Instructions:

Preheat oven to 350°F. Line an 8"x8" baking dish with parchment paper and set aside.

In a standing mixer fitted with a paddle attachment, cream butter and sugar until light and fluffy, about 3 minutes. Add in egg and vanilla during last minute of mixing. Turn mixer speed to low and mix in flour, baking soda, and salt until just combined. Remove from standing mixer and fold in chocolate chips.

Place dough into baking dish and smooth using the back of a spatula. Bake for 30 minutes, or until the top is golden brown and a knife inserted in the center of the dough comes out mostly clean. Allow to cool for 20 minutes before removing from pan and cutting into 9 squares!

Egg Fast Recipe | Eggs Florentine

Ingredients:

- 2 large eggs
- 1 tablespoon unfiltered extra virgin olive oil
- 5 tablespoons Egg Fast Alfredo Sauce (about 1/3 cup)
- 1 tablespoon Organic Parmigiano Regiano Wedge, divided
- 3-grams organic baby spinach
- 1 pinch red pepper flakes

Instructions:

Place oven rack on the top level closest to the broiler. Preheat broiler.

Heat nonstick skillet with olive oil over medium high heat. Add eggs. Fry eggs gently, over medium heat, until whites are mostly set but still raw near the yolk (about 3-4 minutes). Do not flip eggs too easy over. Meanwhile, prepare the casserole.

Spray individual casserole pan with olive oil cooking spray—or drizzle with olive oil. Place half the Alfredo sauce into the bottom of the casserole. Gently slide almost-done-eggs on top of sauce. Top eggs with remaining Alfredo and a 1/2 tablespoon of Parmesan cheese. Place casserole under broiler and broil until the eggs have set and top is golden in spots and bubbly (about 2-3 minutes). Remove and top with julienne (thinly sliced) baby spinach leaves, remaining Parmesan and a pinch of red pepper flakes. Serve immediately to rave reviews!

NOTES

If you've never tried eating garlic and Alfredo sauce for breakfast, you should drop everything you're doing right now and do it immediately. This dish is so good, you'll finish first, then look covetously at your partner's dish and beg for more with your eyes. Whoever came up with using cream and Parmesan with eggs was GENIUS! BTW, remember this works great as an Egg Fast Dish. It's super low carb, the spinach contributes 1g of carbs to the dish and is basically there for color and appeal. Egg Fast Eggs Florentine would be perfect at any meal. (Oh and the Alfredo takes less than 2 minutes to make from start to finish!)

Serving Ideas Serve on its own with a cup of hot coffee or tea, or pair with a small green salad with vinaigrette for an elegant and satisfying meal.

Nutritional Information

Per Serving: 529

Calories; 49g

Fat (82.7% calories from fat); 20g

Protein; 3g

Carbohydrate; trace Dietary

Fiber; 3g

Effective Carbs

Savory Vegetable Crumble (Vegan and Gluten Free)

5 min preparation time

40 min cook time

45 min total time

Ingredients:

- 2 tablespoons olive oil
- 1 small eggplant, cut into 2-inch pieces
- 1 zucchini, cut into 2-inch pieces
- 1 small fennel bulb, sliced thinly
- 1 leek, sliced
- 2 roma tomatoes, chopped
- 2 garlic cloves, minced
- ½ teaspoon dry thyme
- For the crumble:
- ¼ cup garbanzo bean flour
- ¼ cup gluten-free rolled oats
- 2 Tablespoons GO VEGGIE vegan parmesan, plus more for serving
- 1 lemon, zested
- 2 tablespoons olive oil

Instructions:

Heat your oven to 350°F.

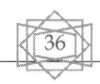

Heat the oil in a large, oven-proof skillet over medium-high heat. Add the eggplant, zucchini, leek, and fennel; cook 10 minutes, or until soft. Add the garlic, tomatoes, and thyme. Season with salt and pepper.

In a small bowl, combine the flour, oats, parmesan, and lemon zest. Stir in the olive oil until everything is combined and all of the dry ingredients are moistened. Sprinkle over the vegetables in an even layer.

Transfer the pan to the oven and bake for 30 minutes, or until the top of the crumble is browned and crisp.

Serve with additional parmesan, as desired.

Notes

If you don't have an oven-proof skillet, transfer the cooked vegetables to a pie plate after step 2.

Gluten Free Pumpkin Pie Hand Pies

Recipe type: Dessert

Cuisine: American

Prep time: 60 mins

Cook time: 15 mins

Total time: 1 hour 15 mins

Serves: 12

Gluten free Pumpkin hand pies, perfect pick up pies great for potlucks and big dinners.

Ingredients:

- Gluten Free Pie Dough
- 2 cups gluten free flour (see notes for brand)
- 1 teaspoon salt
- 1 teaspoon sugar
- 12 tablespoons butter
- 2 eggs
- 4-6 tablespoons iced cold water

Instructions

Place flour, salt, sugar in food processor.

Mix well.

Add in butter. Mix just until the butter is in pea sized pieces.

Add eggs. Mix for about 5 seconds until eggs are incorporated.

Add just enough water to bring together.

Dough will be like a short bread dough, because there is no elastic.

Refrigerate for 30 minutes. It's easier to work with cold.

Flour surface and roll out. Sometimes the gluten free dough will split or break apart a little. Just put it back together. It will stick back together much easier than gluten dough.

Cut 4 inch circles with a biscuit cutter.

Imprint with a decorative stamp if you have one. If not make sure to put a slit into the top to let the steam escape.

Brush milk over the first round.

Put about 2 teaspoons of pumpkin filling onto one round.

Top and gently press the edges together.

Bake at 400 degrees F for 15 minutes on baking dish. I have used both parchment paper and just a baking stone. Both worked fine.

Cool Completely.

These freeze well in plastic freezer bags.

Gluten free super-fast sweet potato "steaks"

Prep Time: 5 minutes

Cook Time: 15 minutes

Total Time: 20 minutes

Yield: 1 Sweet Potato

Ingredients:

- 1 Sweet Potato
- Oil
- Salt and pepper

Instructions:

Peel the skin off of the sweet potato and discard.

Slice the potato into 1/2" thick slices (you can slice them lengthwise for a larger steak or you can make rounds by slicing them crosswise).

Rub all sides of your slices with oil, then season with salt and pepper.

Place on your panini griddle and cook on medium setting for 15 minutes or until soft. You may need to flip the slices half way through cooking time, especially if your slices are of varying thickness.

Notes

Time may vary depending on the panini maker you use.

Gluten-Free Apple-Spice Muffins

Ingredients

- 2 cups almond flour
- 1 teaspoon baking soda
- 4 eggs
- 1 cup unsweetened apple sauce
- 4 tablespoons melted butter
- 1 tablespoon pure vanilla extract
- 1 tablespoon ground cinnamon
- 1 teaspoon ground allspice
- 1 teaspoon ground cloves
- ½ teaspoon kosher salt

How to Make This Recipe:

Preheat the oven to 350°. In a large mixing bowl, thoroughly combine all of the ingredients. Pour the batter equally into a paper-lined muffin tin. They should be approximately three-fourths full.

Bake for 15 minutes, rotating the pan halfway through. Remove from the oven and let cool for five minutes, before removing the muffins from the pan to a wire rack. Serve warm.

Gluten Free Banana Pancakes

Ingredients:

- ½ cup rolled oats
- ½ cup almond flour
- ½ teaspoon baking powder
- a good pinch of sea salt
- 1 medium banana, ripe (about 2/3 cups mashed)
- 2/3 cup plain almond milk

Instructions:

Place all of the ingredients in a blender and puree until smooth. Heat a skillet over medium low heat. When heated, drop a quarter teaspoon of coconut oil in the pan, followed by ¼ cup of pancake batter. Cook for 3 to 4 minutes before flipping (these take a bit longer than traditional pancakes to cook) and an additional 3 to 4 minutes on the other side too. Complete with the rest of the batter, adding a pinch of coconut oil to the pan between pancakes. Keep warm under a towel on a plate until ready to serve.

We enjoy ours with a little drizzle of maple syrup and fresh berries. Coconut ribbons are always welcome too. But dress yours up as you'd like! A slather of nut butter and a dollop of coconut whipped cream would be amazing.

Healthy Chocolate Crepes {Gluten and Grain Free}

Ingredients:
- For the crepes:
- 2 eggs
- 1 banana
- 1 tablespoon cocoa
- For the filling:
- ¼ cup whipped cream (no added sugar)
- 6 oz Greek yogurt
- Optional: 1 tsp stevia
- Toppings:
- Raspberries
- Shaved chocolate

Instructions:
For the crepes:

Add all of the ingredients into a blender or food processor and blend until smooth.

Pour on a hot pan (over medium heat) and cook up until you can flip it and it's not too runny. Cook on the other side for another minute. Keep warm in the oven until they're all made up.

For the filling:

The cream will already be whipped, if you haven't' done that - do that now.

Fold in the Greek yogurt to the whipped cream mixed, add stevia if needed.

Putting it together:

Spoon a few tablespoons into the crepe and wrap up. Top with raspberries and shaved chocolate.

Gluten Free Lemon Chicken Chinese-Style

Ingredients:
- ½ cup freshly squeezed lemon juice (juice from 2 lemons)
- ¼ cup gluten free tamari or soy sauce
- ¼ cup (55 g) packed light brown sugar
- Zest from 1 lemon
- ½ teaspoon ground ginger
- 2/3 cup low sodium chicken stock
- 2 tablespoons (18 g) cornstarch
- 1 egg, beaten with 1 tablespoon water
- Cornstarch, for dredging (about ¾ cup)
- ½ teaspoon garlic salt (optional)
- 1½ pounds boneless, skinless chicken breasts, cut into 1-inch square pieces
- ¼ - ½ cup neutral oil, for frying (canola works well)

Directions:
In a heavy-bottom, medium-size saucepan, place the lemon juice, tamari or soy sauce, brown sugar, lemon zest and ground ginger, and whisk to combine well. Pour about half of the chicken stock into a small bowl, whisk the 2 tablespoons cornstarch into the stock until it is smooth and pour into the saucepan. Pour the remaining chicken stock into the saucepan as well, and whisk to combine well. Set the saucepan aside.

Place the egg and water mixture in a medium bowl. Place the cornstarch for dredging in a separate, medium bowl. Add the garlic salt to the cornstarch, and whisk to combine. Dredge the chicken pieces through the egg wash, then dip in the cornstarch to coat lightly. Shake off any excess. I like to dredge all of the chicken at once before I begin to cook it, so I place the coated chicken on a baking sheet lined with parchment paper along the way.

In a wok or a large, heavy-bottom sauté pan, place about 1/4-inch of frying oil over medium heat until shimmering. Add the chicken in batches and fry until crisp – for about 2-3 minutes total, turning once. Do not crowd the pan. The chicken will not brown, but it will crisp. Remove and drain on paper towels. Add more oil as necessary.

To make the sauce, place the saucepan with the lemon/soy mixture over medium heat, and bring to a boil. Lower the heat to medium-low and cook, whisking constantly until thickened (about 3 minutes). Toss the chicken in the sauce, and serve immediately over rice.

Gluten Free Coconut Cream Cheesecake

Prep Time: 15 minutes

Cook Time: 1 hour, 30 minutes

Total Time: 1 hour, 45 minutes

Yield: 16 slices

Serving Size: 1 slice

Calories per serving: 401

Fat per serving: 37.9g

Cheesecake is one of the most popular low carb high fat desserts. We love this yummy gluten free coconut cream cheesecake. A great way to fill up on fat!

Ingredients:
CRUST:
- 1 ½ cups almond flour
- 1 teaspoon cinnamon
- 3 tablespoons sweetener (I used Swerve)
- ½ cup butter, melted

FILLING:
- 4 (8 oz) boxes cream cheese, softened
- ¾ cup sweetener (I used Swerve)
- ½ of 13.5 oz canned coconut cream (200ml)
- 3 large eggs
- 1 teaspoon vanilla extract

FROSTING:
- ½ of 13.5 oz canned coconut cream (200ml)
- ¼ cup powdered sweetener (I used Sukrin Melis)
- 2 tablespoons cream cheese, softened

Instructions:

Mix together crust ingredients and press into the bottom of a spring form pan. Refrigerate while preparing filling.

In a large bowl, beat together filling ingredients. Mix just until smooth.

Pour filling onto the crust and bake at 350°F for 15 minutes. Reduce the heat to 250°F and bake for another 75-90 minutes.

Allow to cool completely in the refrigerator. Run knife along edge of cake and remove springform side.

For frosting, beat together coconut cream, powdered sugar, and cream cheese until creamy.

Spread frosting over the cooled cake. Refrigerate for at least an hour before slicing.

Notes

Makes 16 slices

Nutrition per slice: 401 calories, 37.9g fat, 297mg sodium, 4.9g carbs, 1.2g fiber, 3.7g net carbs, 8.2g protein, 4.3g erythritol

Gluten-free potato croquettes

Ingredients:
- 450g potatoes
- ½ tablespoon butter
- 1 egg yolk
- 2 tablespoons hot milk
- Salt & pepper
- 75g gluten free flour
- 1 egg
- 60g gluten free breadcrumbs

Instructions:
1. Pass 450g boiled, mashed potatoes through wire sieve, return to pan, beat in 1/2 tablespoon butter, 1 egg yolk, 2 tablespoons hot milk and season with salt and pepper.
2. Divide into cork-shaped pieces and roll in gluten free seasoned flour (seasoned with salt and pepper), then brush with beaten egg and roll in fine gluten free breadcrumbs.
3. Fry in deep fat fryer until golden brown. (Frying oil should not have been previously used for any foods that may not be gluten free)

Made in the USA
Middletown, DE
28 November 2020